Healing with Music and Color

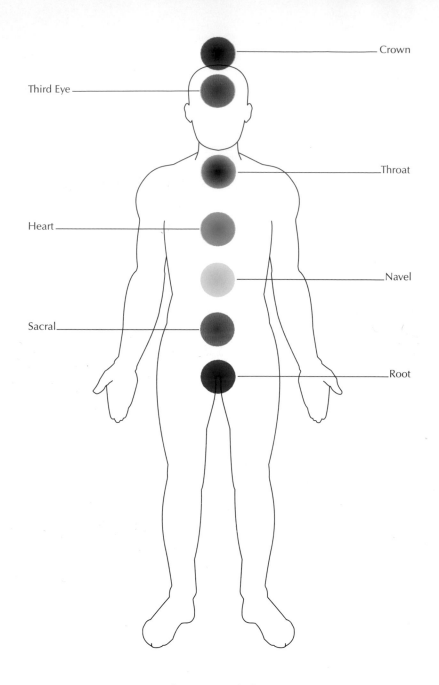

Crown

Third Eye

Throat

Heart

Navel

Sacral

Root

The Seven Chakras

HEALING
with Music and Color

A BEGINNER'S GUIDE

by
Mary Bassano

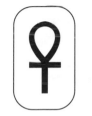

SAMUEL WEISER, INC.

York Beach, Maine

First published in 1992 by
Samuel Weiser, Inc.
Box 612
York Beach, ME 03910

Library of Congress Cataloging-in-Publication Data

Bassano, Mary, 1916–
    Healing with music and color : a beginner's guide /
Mary Bassano.
      p.   cm.
    Includes bibliographical references.
    1. Vital force--Therapeutic use.   2. Color--
Therapeutic use.   3. Sound--Therapeutic use.   I. Title.
RZ999.B27 1992
615.8'3--dc20   92–16857
                                                CIP

ISBN 0-87728-760-0
BJ

Printed in the United States of America

The paper used in this publication meets the minimum
requirements of the American National Standard for Per-
manence of Paper for Printed Library Materials
Z39.48–1984.

Dedicated to Jean, a special
person and a special friend.

Contents

Acknowledgments viii

Chapter 1 – Philosophy and Background 1

Chapter 2 – You Are a Musical Instrument 9

Chapter 3 – Colors and the Aura 19

Chapter 4 – Red 27

Chapter 5 – Orange 35

Chapter 6 – Yellow 41

Chapter 7 – Green 45

Chapter 8 – Blue 51

Chapter 9 – Indigo 57

Chapter 10 – Violet 63

Chapter 11 – Pastels and Iridescences 69

Chapter 12 – Manifesting Universal Energies
             with Crystals 73

Chapter 13 – Techniques 85

Chapter 14 – Conclusion 97

Glossary 101

Bibliography 103

About the Author 105

Acknowledgments

My heartfelt thanks to all those who have helped me in so many ways, especially: Virginia Dory, for her excellent editing and helpful suggestions; Dr. Millard Walker, for his help and suggestions along the way; Marion L. Peterson, for correcting and typing the manuscript; Roberta Herzog, for her initial help and continued encouragement; and finally, Murial McCord and my many good friends, for their continual support and encouragement.

Chapter One

PHILOSOPHY AND BACKGROUND

Let us picture the beginning of our great creation, seeing it as a mass of energy, whirling, rotating, vibrating until worlds, planets and stars were formed. All universes were filled with these energies which radiated forth from the creative sound of the One Divine Source, bringing with it universal light.

Tones and colors eventually evolved, all having a direct relationship with each other. Emanations from these sound and color spectra filled the planets, giving each its own individual energy which, down through the ages, has cast its influence on mankind. When the planets move in their orbits, each emits its own tone and radiates its own color. Those who are clairvoyant and clairaudient may often perceive these beautiful and powerful energies.

The Universe is One, and we see that there is an intermingling and relatedness not only with things on Earth, but, even more significantly, with influences from the outer universe, and with each human being.

As we read now about these marvelous healing energies available to us, let us keep in mind that we, too, are participating in this ever ongoing spectacular drama of life—all as a result of that first Creative Sound. How great and powerful it must have been to have brought forth such magnificence! And God said, "Let there be Light and there was light."[1]

As Light radiated forth, it broke up into seven component parts, each being directed by Spirit to its appropriate center or chakra, in each individual. These seven colors, or Spirits of Light as they are sometimes termed, are the colors of the spectrum. They enter our being through the magnetic field surrounding and radiating from our seven bodies—physical and subtle. There are more colors than the spectrum seven, of course; additional chakras in the body, and possibly other and higher invisible bodies. However, for the purpose of this text, we will work with the most generally accepted seven colors and chakras.

These seven colors also have a correlation with the seven-note diatonic scale which is regarded as standard in our Western culture. It has been determined, according to the Pythagorean theory of color and music, that there are comparable vibrational frequencies between the seven spectrum colors and the seven-note scale, both within the whole tones and half tones. Red vibrates to middle C, Orange to D, Yellow to E, Green to F (half step), Blue to G, Indigo to A and Violet to B.[2] (See Table 1 on pages 4–5.)

The seven pure spectrum colors relate to the middle octave of the keyboard. However, there are continuing relationships between the treble and bass octaves with

---

[1]All biblical references are from The King James Bible (Nashville, TN: Thomas Nelson, 1976), Genesis 1:3.
[2]Manly P. Hall, *The Secret Teachings of All Ages* (Los Angeles, CA: Philosophical Research Society, 1975), p. lxxxiv.

various shading of the spectrum colors. The colors relating to the octave *below* the middle octave would be deeper and darker, but with the same tonal correlation. For example, the C below middle C would still be in the red family, but would be deeper than the red of middle C. The tones *above* the middle octave would be represented by lighter and more luminous colors.

Everything in the universe responds to light and tone. This includes both animal and vegetable life. Every human being, including each of its atoms and cells, responds to that being's own particular key note and color vibration. Therefore, learning an individual's tone and color can aid in applying the proper energies for that person. In recognizing the fact that color and music emanate genuine energy frequencies, we know that we can use facets of these energies for healing and for ever greater spiritual awareness. They can be used most effectively when we understand the qualities contained in each color and each musical tone. (Please refer to the chapters on the various colors and to Table 1, pages 4–5, to understand these relationships and characteristics.)

Just what is this therapy and why and how does it work? The art or science of color and music therapy is an ancient one. It was known to the sages of old and is now being revealed once again to us in this Aquarian Age. Eons ago, color and music were used for healing in Greece and Egypt; the ancient civilizations of India and China were also aware of the therapeutic value of color and music. Rather than having hospitals as we have today, they had temples that served as resting and spiritually

Table 1. Seven Synergetic Energies and Their Uses.

Colors	Tones	Chakras	Glands	Physical & Subtle Bodies
Red	C	Root (Base of Spine)	Ovaries Gonads	Physical
Orange	D	Sacral	Spleen Liver	Etheric
Yellow	E	Navel	Adrenals Pancreas	Astral
Green	F	Heart	Thymus	Lower Mental
Blue	G	Throat	Thyroid	Higher Mental
Indigo	A	Third Eye	Pituitary	Spiritual
Violet	B	Crown	Pineal	Divine Monad

Table 1. (continued).

Characteristics	Healing for
Physical strength, leadership, independence	Anemia, poor circulation, lack of energy
Self-respect, courage, the introvert	Low blood pressure, nerves, fear
The introvert, the thinker, emotional, good intellect	Stomach disorders, depression, slow learning, nerves
Balance, tranquillity, healing ability	Heart, circulation, ulcers, imbalances
Coolness, calmness, peace, God-centered, purifier	High blood pressure, fevers, skin problems, tension, internal infections, cancer
Intuition, dedication, cleanser, memory ability, communication with other worlds, violet	Nervous disorders, problems with medications, lack of motivation, some mental and nervous disorders
Dedication, surrender to the "I AM" path of service, awareness of one's divinity	Feeling of unworthiness, lack of motivation, some mental and nervous disorders

energizing places where these healing techniques were applied.[3]

Color and music serve not merely to heal but also to remove blocks within the individual so that the *natural* energies can be allowed to do their perfect work in the healing process. We are now relearning some of this ancient wisdom and implementing it with an ever greater awareness and knowledge that is being revealed to us in this new and accelerated age.

This therapy works because we, as spiritual beings, are highly susceptible to both positive and negative effects of vibratory influences in our everyday lives, although we are often unaware of this. We are affected by the *differences* in vibrations. For example, looking at bright red, wearing it, feeling it, elicits one sensation. Wearing blue or being in a room with a lot of that color brings another entirely different response. Therefore, by learning the qualities of each color and finding music that relates to the energy and mood of the color, we can use these tools constructively. (Music suggestions are given at the end of each "color" chapter.) Sound and light affect everyone to some extent, but it is ever true that the more awareness we have, the greater will be the response.

Color and music can also be considered non-verbal forms of communication. When we know a person's basic tone and color ray, we can tap into that energy with these tools and establish a rapport with the individual. The person being treated then realizes that the therapist understands his or her feelings; there is communication and the treatment can begin. Also, playing certain compositions of music can speak volumes to the listening ear. The music

---

[3]Roland Hunt, *The Seven Keys to Colour Healing* (Saffron Walden, England: C. W. Daniel, 1971), p. 17.

communicates as with colors. Being able to relate to someone on his or her own wave length is very necessary when working with anyone. (Please refer to chapter thirteen, "Techniques," for information on determining people's basic note and color.)

The modalities can affect us on all levels once we comprehend which musical rhythms, harmonies and tonalities can energize the body, stimulate the mind, calm the emotions and be most effective in raising the spiritual consciousness.

The same principle applies to colors. As an example, one color may be excellent for stimulating the brain cells, another may be better for developing the intuitive sense, and still a third will be more applicable in bringing peace and quietness to the mind.

Color and music may be used separately, of course, but when the two are used together the vibrational energy increases and brings added healing strengths to the individual being treated. Also, it helps to sensitize the individual on whom the music and color is focused, so that he or she becomes more aware of sounds and tones *within* color and of colors within musical notes and compositions.

The philosophy, as expressed in this book, should be applicable in all phases of our lives, leading us to recognize the Oneness in all things, in tones, in colors, and in all of nature. Once we know the power of our thoughts, we can use our minds to create and direct these energies in a positive and healing way.

Chapter Two

YOU ARE A MUSICAL INSTRUMENT

We are all instruments of one kind or another, but we are also entire symphonies. Our bodies are constantly radiating colors and their corresponding tones, depending at any moment on our state of health and emotional and spiritual consciousness. So, considering ourselves as instruments, how are we playing at any given time? Are we aware of the depth of our feelings as we play the cello, or are we irritated and angry as we pound the drums? We may be at peace and filled with Light as we produce flute-like tones from our very self.

We are instruments, but we are also an entire symphony. As we bring all the emotions, spiritual awareness, and physical energies into play, are we not creating a symphony of sounds? Not only sounds, but rhythms enter into the compositions we have created and are now creating. As we are playing our melodies and harmonies, so is all life. Are we not, then, contributing in some small part to the music of the spheres? The planets, too, hum their tones as they revolve around the Sun, and they, also, are a part of this majestic whole. When we are experiencing good health, there is a continuous sound, somewhat like the hum of the bumble bee that proceeds forth from the vital body. The keynote of this vital body is in harmony with the keynote of the archetype.

Every form, whether it be human, plant, or animal, emits its own special sound and, likewise, every sound radiates a certain color. The two are inextricably intertwined. *Sound is audible color and color is visible sound.* "Every organ of man's body-temple has been fashioned by the creative rhythms of the starry hierarchies. The beating of the heart, the flow of the blood, the play of the muscles, the pulsations of the breath are all a part of this great body-symphony."[1]

When we attempt to tune an instrument—a violin, for example—we listen to the strings as we draw the bow across them. We must learn to distinguish the subtleties of discords and fine tuning. Gradually, through practice, we become attuned to our inner selves. We turn the peg, "strings" become aligned, and we are then in tune with the cosmic sounds and with our own soul.

Meditation is, of course, one of the ways in which we may tune up our strings. By relaxing, letting go, and becoming one with the Universal Spirit, we can feel our centers gaining balance, our thoughts and emotions becoming quiet. Music that is inspiring and uplifting, along with related colors, can help to bring this fine tuning of the spirit.

Music is the most subtle of the art forms but probably has the greatest influence on our psychic centers and sympathetic nervous system. It also may affect the parasympathetic or automatic nervous system either directly or indi-

---

[1]Corinne Heline, *Healing and Regeneration Through Music* (Santa Barbara, CA: J. F. Rowny Press, 1965), p. 9.

rectly. The entire universe is undoubtedly vibrating to certain frequencies, and we are influenced by them according to our own nerve responses.

Undoubtedly, all physical ailments have their own rate of vibrations, too, and if this could be measured, then tones with a sympathetic vibration could be applied with beneficial results. One day this "measuring" will be possible. It might seem that an opposing vibration—rather than a sympathetic one—would be required. However, the physical explanation is that the sound vibration sets up a *comparable* frequency with another object or person. The vibration of that person or object is unable to tolerate the stress of a *similar* vibration. It is as though the "darkness," or physical illness, could not endure the healthy vibration or, in a sense, could not accept the light, and so the imbalance would dissolve or break away. It is commonly told that Caruso, by singing a certain high note, caused a glass to break. This would indicate that the note he sang was sympathetic to the vibration of the glass, which could not stand that frequency of sound.

Since this chapter is primarily about music, let's find ways in which this particular tool can be used effectively. All our great composers have been attuned to cosmic forces, to the devic kingdom and to the Illumined Ones. Since they have received inspiration from these sources, their music reflects these energies and spiritual vibrations. It is said that the music of Scriabin, Debussy, Wagner, and Bartok has been inspired by the nature devas, and much of this (and other music, as well) can help open up the spiritual centers.

By being honest with ourselves, we can determine what areas of our being need help. For instance, if your emotions are out of control, you should know there is a need to balance the solar plexus area, and so you would try to find music that will calm, balance, and *lift* the emotional responses. If perhaps, you are "spaced out" a good deal of the time, and your feet are not touching the ground, then you know that the lower chakras must be balanced along with the pineal and pituitary. Likewise, if you are engrossed in the physical and material, then you must find music to activate the higher centers. To energize these spiritual chakras, we should continue to listen to ourselves, so that we may find those discordant strings and use our spiritual tuning forks to work on ourselves.

Both Earth and people alternate between major and minor moods, corresponding to major and minor keys in music. The minor keys help us develop subjectivity (the inner self) and the major ones impel us to be outgoing and creative. Music that is primarily rhythmic affects the physical body; music which is essentially melodic deals with the emotions; and the harmonics of music relate to spiritual energies.

Let us consider the *physical* first. Strong rhythms, loud sound, and discordant tones can stir the physical senses, shatter glass, and destroy matter. For instance, soldiers marching on a suspension bridge must break their marching rhythms to an uneven step or the sustained rhythm could cause the bridge to collapse. Consider the rhythmic and hypnotic dances that become so energized as to project people into trances and excite sexual urges. Martial and patriotic music, although strongly rhythmic, can have positive effects—such as energizing a lethargic person, stimulating circulation, or giving vitality to the physical body. Retarded people are usually helped more by a steady, well-structured rhythm than by a smooth flowing melody.

We see rhythm in all phases of Nature. "Winds are tuned to certain rhythms, as is also the beat of the waves.

The tides also have their rhythms, coming in on majors and going out on minors. . . . The combined sounds of everything on earth compose a harmonic chord which is the keynote of our planet. It is in the key of F whose tone becomes visible as green, nature's basic color . . ."[2]

On the *emotional* level, music with a clear melody reaches the feeling nature—it helps us release tension and enables us to search ourselves in regard to emotions and feelings. It aids our ability to express and become creative.

On the *spiritual* level, the harmonies of music seem to reach deeper, touching the higher Self. Music with deep, meaningful harmony can lift us to a higher level of consciousness. In the inner realms, we can learn to listen to our own sound and tune into pure spirit for direction and guidance.

In addition to different kinds of music, let us be aware of the various instruments, each with its own special sounds and vibrational frequencies. An oboe can elicit a certain response; the violin quite a different feeling. So each instrument by itself can have a specific value, depending on our need for or response to it.

Melody and harmony follow after rhythm in the development of music, evolving as our awareness and sensitivity evolved. As we became more and more cognizant of the Higher Self, music evolved that can reach the inner person. The degree to which we hear the *soul* of music—the sound within the sound—is the measure of our God awareness. The music to which we relate reflects *us*. We may change the "you" that is projected by involving ourselves in different music that can bring about desired

[2]Horatio Costa, "New Age Music, Cosmic Sounds, and the Music of the Spheres," *The American Theosophist* (Wheaton, IL: Theosophical Society of America, May/June 1989), p. 65.

changes. Certain sounds and tones can change the very chemistry of our bodies, and can lift a low emotional state to an altered state of consciousness, thereby tuning up the instrument that is each of us.

As mentioned previously, it would appear that music evolves as we evolve. Nations and cultures are reflected in their music. However, from another point of view, Cyril Scott, who received channeled teachings from the Master, Koot Hoomi, said, "An innovation in musical style has invariably been followed by an innovation in politics and morals. The decline of music in early Egypt and Greece was followed by the complete decline of the Egyptian and Grecian civilizations themselves."[3] He further states that music is a more powerful force in the molding of character than religious creeds or moral philosophers, and that there is always an indirect, if not direct, influence of music on people. So it is questionable whether a change in society and politics comes first and then the resultant music, or whether music changes are produced first, thus affecting cultural and sociological changes. There are always differences of opinion in any philosophical premise, but by studying history and our continual evolvement, we may someday arrive at the truth.

In working with music, it is very helpful to know your key note. Once you have found your tone, you should make proper use of it by intoning or playing in that key to achieve total balance. Intoning the AUM sound on your personal note can exert a very powerful effect on your entire being—on all levels.

Recognizing that every person and every object has its own key note can account for a blending of personalities.

---

[3]Cyril Scott, *Music: Its Secret Influence Throughout the Ages* (London: Aquarian Press, 1958), p. 42.

If the notes produce a discord, then there is a disharmony between those individuals or objects. "When humanity shall have developed clairaudience together with the ability to determine the keynote of any person or thing, then friends, places and positions will be selected in accordance with basic tonal compatibility."[4]

From the ancient wisdom teachings, we learn that the sages of old knew how to determine the individual's key note and its related planet. Then those energies could be used for a "tuning up" of the "instrument." This knowledge is still available to those who tune in to the Higher Self and learn to listen intuitively.

From many of the Edgar Cayce readings, we learn that the Atlantean civilization was very advanced and used music that was probably a combination of Oriental and Occidental influences. Cayce also reported that a form of electricity was known in this culture. It had very high vibrations and this electrical energy was used in various healing techniques. The music of ancient India was, according to Cayce, in quarter tones, which were used in chants and produced a high state of consciousness.[5] To us, these quarter tones would seem to be off pitch. In comparing music, we learn that the music of ancient Egypt was usually in third tones—which aided mental development rather than spiritual.

So many of these ancient cultures knew and made use of color, music, and other forms of art in the process of spiritual development. Much of this heritage was lost for a time and is now being brought back to our remembrance with, hopefully, additional knowledge and tools for healing and modern spiritual growth.

---

[4]Corinne Heline, *Healing and Regeneration*, p. 11.
[5]Edgar Cayce, *Readings: The Searchlight* (Virginia Beach, VA: A.R.E., Dec. 1960), p. 2.

However, not only do *ancient* cultures differ, but also present cultures have different tonal systems. Many tonal scales are recognized early in infancy (maybe before birth—intrauterine). However, there are also groupings of notes or melodies that are considered almost universal. Therefore, we must learn to appreciate where and when these differences occur and make necessary adjustments in our approach to music therapy so that music can, indeed, continue to be the "language of the soul."

It is said that music has power to soothe the savage beast, and, as we know, the biblical David used music therapy in calming King Saul by playing his harp. Today, we know much more about the healing properties of music.

The use of music on the thymus gland is another example of these healing energies. This gland is very important in governing the life energy of the body. Therefore, since music has such great potential for stimulating the life forces, we should apply it, along with color, to aid the functioning of the thymus. The thymus gland is a link between the mind and body. So, as we focus the music/color energies in that direction, we will be able to balance and energize this mind-body connection.

Sound obviously has a tremendous power which was understood by the Masters of old. There are many references to this. One example is the leveling of the walls of Jericho mentioned in the Bible. For six days men marched around the city, blowing on rams' horns. On the seventh day the men blew a loud blast in unison and the walls collapsed. Most importantly, as we consider *sound*, the world was created in the beginning by God speaking the word, or the creative sound.

We can utilize so much classical and New Age music in our healing that we should familiarize ourselves with these tools that are available to us. What music stirs your creative spark? What tones bring peace to your soul? Can you communicate through music? Then *use* the tones and compositions that express you and let those wonderful energies fill you and overwhelm you with their beauty and healing.

As we enter the next phase of our planet's evolution, music and color both will undoubtedly play a very significant part. A more peaceful and spiritually uplifting atmosphere will prevail, just as soon as more people become attuned to these higher vibrations of healing and balance.

Chapter Three
_____

COLORS AND THE AURA

Beautiful colors and beautiful music both have a very significant impact on our lives. Colors have an affect above and beyond visual responses. Imagine yourself being led—blindfolded—and with all external and sensory stimuli being absent, into a room with cheery, vibrant colors. Then, in the same manner, feel yourself being led into a prison cell with drab, colorless walls and furniture. Would you feel the difference in these two rooms, regardless of the fact that you could not see? Yes. Colors, as well as everything else in the world, emit vibrational frequencies that reach you in various ways.

You feel, hear, and see with many parts of your body. The very cells in your skin can pick up auditory or visual vibrations without the use of ears and eyes. Helen Keller is a marvellous example of this. One way in which she was able to "see" and experience a dance program was by placing her hands on the floor and *feeling* the vibrations and rhythms of the dancers.

Blind people can learn to see colors by touching; the fingers develop a sensitivity that can distinguish these differences. Experiments have been conducted in Bulgaria using the Soviet technique of "skin sight." The children chosen for this testing were blind from birth or early infancy. Many of them were immediately able to distinguish colors and geometrical figures by skin sight. Other blind children were also able to detect colors and figures after some training.[1]

As you examine the deeper, esoteric meaning of color, you will realize that the use of various colors can help to lift spiritual consciousness, can quiet the emotions, and can actually bring psychic benefits to the body. You can literally change your world by making better use of (and becoming more aware of) the wonderful color energies that are available.

The seven spectrum colors are used as basic tools in the color therapist's work. However, there are blendings of these colors, such as turquoise (blue and green), magenta (purple and red), amethyst, coral and peach. These blended shades can also be very beneficial.

It is necessary to consider the off spectrum colors, such as brown, beige, gray and black as well. These often indicate fear, insecurity, a need to hide from the world, and, frequently, materialism.

Certain beige and grays, when combined with silver or rose tones, *can*, at times, be used to advantage, as the negative effect of a completely dark color would be less. A dull gray or beige, however, can have a very depressing and depleting effect. A warm, rich brown often indicates good human relationships and an affinity with the earth, whereas a dull brown may signify a materialistic attitude.

Black is sometimes the choice made when you are turning inward—perhaps while a new idea is being born. All things germinate first in darkness. However, every-

---

[1]Sheila Ostrander and Lynn Schroeder, *Psychic Discoveries Behind the Iron Curtain*, (Englewood Cliffs, NJ: Prentice Hall, 1970), p. 290.

thing comes out into the light eventually. Black can also indicate a need to hide, either from yourself or others. If this is your chosen color, it may mean that you are not accepting the responsibilities on your "agreed upon" path in life.

These dark colors are not always harmful or negative, however. They may be serving a useful purpose. Occasionally, people of very high spiritual consciousness may wear plain, dark colors. This may be done in order to "ground" these spiritually high people. Dark colors can also be used by hypertense individuals who need to tone down the nervous system. We all need grounding at times, and the dark colors may bring balance at a particular moment. Individual evaluation is most necessary. People should not make flat statements, such as, "black is bad," and "blue is beautiful." The exclusive use of any one color, however, should be recognized as being significant in showing imbalances.

Considering the lights of the spectrum, black is the absence of all such colors; white is the perfect balancing of these lights. White may always be used for protection, healing, and spiritual illumination. In many instances, though, more energy of one specific color may be needed. Therefore, each color plays its part and is necessary to the whole. It has been said that eons ago we saw only four colors—red, black, white, and yellow. Now, as human beings advance, we are able to see many more because as our inner awareness increases, so does our vision develop.

An explanation of the various spectrum colors has been given in chapter one and, in more detail, in the chapters on each specific color. Also refer to the chart for comparisons.

In considering the aura, let us see it as an interblending of color energies radiating from our various bodies. The aura which is most readily seen is from the etheric body. This "body" is often referred to as the "etheric double," as it is not a body of itself but is a "carbon copy," we might say, of the physical. It is also called the health aura as it is through this etheric substance that the sun's energies reach our physical bodies, and the color or colors emanating from this etheric body indicate our state of health, if interpreted correctly.

Clairvoyants, who can see more readily than the average person, can view the aura, using it as a diagnostic tool. "Holes" may often be observed, signifying an imbalance of some kind. However, it is not enough merely to see the auric field; one must know how to interpret the colors that appear, and also notice the colors that appear in relationship to the colors that are absent. Healing work can be done on the aura itself, and this can prevent an imbalance from manifesting in the physical body if the work is done in a timely fashion.

Although the color radiations from the etheric body are the most observable, color vibrations also emanate from the astral, mental, and spiritual bodies. These are of such a luminous quality that they are not easily seen. These colors intertwine and change constantly, depending on changes at the mental, physical and emotional level within the individual.

Every human being has a basic color, and it must of necessity remain in the aura during an entire lifetime. Other colors come and go as we each move back and forth in our emotional and physical phases. However, your personal color represents *you* and is always yours. If we could read the aura reflected from the seven bodies of the individual, it would show us the totality of a person's life.

"Concisely speaking, it is a subtle, superphysical emanation surrounding a person in the form of a luminous mist of clouds. . . . It reveals his character, emotional nature, mental caliber, state of health and spiritual development."[2]

Everything in nature radiates an aura. This fact has been scientifically validated by many. Of special importance is the work of Dr. Kilner, who has devised a kind of glass screen through which the aura may be more easily seen. Also of significant importance is the development of Kirlian photography, a method of producing photographs from the action of high-frequency currents, which shows the auras of plants as well as humans.[3] If we are open to reports from those who are truly clairvoyant, then these reports, too, give validation.

The aura is oval in shape and extends beyond the body in direct relationship to our development on all levels. The greater our growth, the larger and more luminous will be the colors of the aura. As we go through the death experience, the aura begins to fade, and it disappears as the silver cord is broken.

We have to be very perceptive when reading an aura as many things must be taken into consideration—the positioning of a color or colors, the intensity and intermingling of the colors, and the dominance of one color over another. All this must be given careful assessment before we can reach an accurate evaluation and diagnosis. By learning the energy characteristics of each color and then developing the ability to *see* the aura, we can determine a great deal about potential, and areas where healing needs to take place. For example, if a bright, clear yellow is

[2]S. C. J. Ousely, *The Power of the Rays* (London: L. N. Fowler, 1951), p. 24.
[3]Stanley Krippner and Daniel Rubin, eds., *The Kirlian Aura* (Garden City, NY: Anchor Press, 1974), p. 35.

observed, it would probably indicate a person with good intellect; a clear blue or violet could signify high spiritual motivation; a murky, muddy red might mean a lustful or materialistic personality.

The auric fields of the various bodies intermingle and are clearly distinguishable through intuitive perception. Not only do the spectrum colors show in the aura, but also blendings of these colors and, often, the off-spectrum colors, such as black, brown, or gray. As mentioned previously, the auric emanations are in constant motion and change constantly as we change.

In trying to see the aura, think of these radiations as being similar to heat waves that you might see shimmering up from the pavement on a hot summer day. If you cannot see the aura but want to know the extent of it, feel with your hands near, but not touching, the physical body, and become aware of energy changes, distance, and heat and cold. If you are adept at using the pendulum, this could be another way of measuring, if not seeing, the aura. Perhaps you can *sense* colors around a person without the aid of the physical eye.

If you wish to try seeing, have someone stand against a clear wall with only a soft light in the room and look at the periphery of the head and shoulders. Don't strain at it. At first you may see just light, but as you work with this concept, you will probably begin to see a change in the color around the individual. This can be developed, if you persevere, but don't try to force it. Let it develop in its own right time. After you become more adept at this, try it in a room with no light at all.

Everything that has life has an aura. And what does not have life, to one degree or another? Learn to look at trees, flowers, and animals as well as looking at people. Begin to allow your inner and outer sight to open wider so you can see the more subtle energies of life. As you grow spiritually and learn to control your emotions and thoughts, your aura will produce beautiful, iridescent and luminous colors, eventually evolving into that pure light of Spirit which is the ultimate goal.

Remember, to those who can see, your aura is showing!

Chapter Four

RED

As we begin to contemplate the wonderful spiritual energies that music and color can give us, let's discover the purpose of each individual color of the spectrum. Also, think about all the great musical compositions, single tones, and various harmonies that can lift us, inspire and actually *change* our beings. Recognizing that color rays and musical tones have a direct, vibratory correspondence with each other, we can then utilize these energies to our benefit—for positive results.

Red, the first color of the spectrum, relates to the first or root chakra, and to the note of C in the middle octave. It represents our life energy—the blood.

The physical stimulation that the color red offers is not comfortable for everybody. For some, it can energize in a positive manner and brings about increased circulation in the body. For others, however, it may be over-stimulating, harsh, and even offensive. We all respond to the stimuli of the moment according to our level of receptivity at that moment. It is natural that there will be different responses to colors and music, even though there are generalities that can be expressed for each one of these energies.

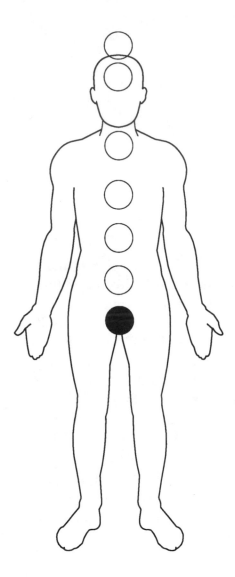

Figure 1. Red relates to the root chakra (the first chakra) at the base of the spine. Through this chakra, the red portion of pure white light enters the body. Both are associated with our physical strength.

If we observe carefully what our bodies and emotions are telling us, we will know what is beneficial for us and what is detrimental. People who respond in a positive way to red would undoubtedly be of high energy and independence. On the other hand, such people might also be repelled because the red would just be adding more "fuel to the fire," giving stimulation where it is not needed, due to the high energy level already within them. It would negate their natural energy to wear more red or to have this color around them.

By the same token, those people who are quite lethargic and/or despondent should not be exposed *immediately* to red as it would be too great a shock to the system. With these people, the color energy should be built up gradually, first reaching them at the present level, then moving on, perhaps with some yellows, then orange, and eventually red, if this is indicated.

Imagine yourself now in a room in which you are completely surrounded by a bright, clear, stimulating red. Visualize the wall, ceiling, rugs and all the furnishings of this red. How do you feel? Now at the same time, put on a record of a Sousa march or something equally strong and rhythmic. If you cannot actually play such a record right now, perhaps you are familiar enough with some march music to hear it with your inner ear. What does this do for you?

At a later time, take a small piece of something red and hold it in your hands, or place it at the bottom of your foot where there are nerve endings. See if you feel energy, but perhaps to a different degree than in the previous experience.

These experiments can help to differentiate between an overabundance or overpowering amount of a certain color, and a mere suggestion of that same energy. It is essential to think of *balance* and *moderation* in any kind of treatment. Red, in particular, because of its extremely strong stimulating power, must be used *very carefully*, and each person to whom you may be giving this red treatment must be evaluated on an individual basis.

This evaluation can be done psychically, with a muscle test (refer to the chapter on techniques) or by applying red to the person and observing the results. If red makes patients feel hot, irritated, and overstimulated, then it is obvious that red is too strong or too harsh for them. On the other hand, if they can feel the vibrations of this energy flowing through, if they experience warmth and strength, then red is right for them.

A "treatment" may consist of applying the needed color with the use of colored light bulbs, drinking color solarized water, using the selected color in home decor or clothing, in color breathing, and/or in visualizing the color surrounding and filling patients completely.

In the chapters on music and techniques, we discuss finding our individual musical tone. In the same way, each of us has a color ray, indicating our path in this lifetime. People on the red path would manifest strong physical energies, independence of character, initiative, and vitality. They would undoubtedly be involved in work of a physical nature. Once people know their basic color and tone, then they have a better understanding of themselves and their potential. Also, they know what additional colors will blend with this individual color. Additional colors can be combined to bring the totality of our being into better balance. The *complimentary* color of our true color ray should be used to help us absorb those qualities that the ray represents.

Since red is primarily a *physical* energizer, let's consider some of the conditions for which this color may be beneficial. Low blood pressure, anemia, arthritis, emphysema, and poor circulation can often be helped by applications of red. A chronic sinus condition, or any problem where there is congestion and/or rigidity may benefit from the use of this penetrating and stimulating color, which can break up and disintegrate calcified deposits and the like. It must be emphasized, however that red is a color which must be used with prudence due to the intensity of its vibrations. Where red *might* be considered, orange or yellow may be the better choice. Again, individual evaluation is most necessary.

Red relates to the root chakras at the base of the spine, or the coccygeal area. (Please refer to the glossary for further clarification.) This is the area through which that particular portion (red) of the pure white light of Spirit enters the body. Each color is an individualization of the universal light and comes to us in varying vibrational frequencies by way of the psychic centers (comparable to the seven main glandular centers) on our bodies, each color relating to a particular center.

An important point to remember is that a color in its particular center may or may not be used for healing in that specific area. Red, for example, being such a stimulating color, would not be used to treat cancer in the gonad area, as it would only encourage growth. However, if this chakra in itself needs stimulation, then its own color (red) could be used. Each color in its representative chakra should be used to motivate *only* when balancing is needed—not to over-energize.

The relationship of red to music is in the key of C or the single note in the middle octave. Intoning in the related tone, playing on an instrument, or listening to a composition in this key can increase the energies when working with a color.

MARCH MILITAIRE

Schubert

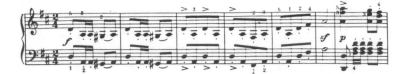

In rare instances, red might be used with someone who has a lot of repressed anger. By using a brief treatment with red, the therapist could establish rapport with such an individual. At the same time, the patient might be helped in expressing his or her concealed anger, as red could act as a triggering aid. After this short application of the red color, a more quiet, more relaxing and, therefore, more supporting color should be given. This type of treatment should be considered only after careful evaluation, while giving much support and acceptance.

We can find relationships of red in Nature — beautifully colored leaves in the fall, lovely red roses, the various shades of red on birds. All of these examples show us some of the many varieties of one basic color, giving us yet another feeling of this color and the many ways the color may be used and developed.

Your responses to color may differ according to your mood, physical health and emotional state. Your emotions and thoughts are as varied as are the shades and hues of colors. How do you respond, for instance, when you look at a beautiful maple leaf that you may observe in the fall of the year, as compared with your response to a vivid red dress that you see hanging on a clothes rack? Do you see red in the sky with, perhaps, its reflections in the water? What part of red do you like and *when* do you like it?

Study your likes and dislikes and your reactions to these varieties of experiences and you will know yourself better.

Red Music

Classical	New Age
March Militaire by Schubert	Mars Music from *The Planets* by Holst
Sousa Marches	*On the Edge* by Micky Hart
The Sailor's Dance from *Red Poppy Ballet Suite* by Gliere	*Diga Rhythm* by Micky Hart

Chapter Five

ORANGE

To experience orange, the second color of the spectrum, feel yourself enveloped in a cocoon-like covering of this color. Let it permeate your being, and try to be aware of your response to it.

This is a warm, invigorating, and nourishing color, and, if used properly, it can revitalize you. Orange, however, like red, may be too stimulating for some individuals as it is a color of high energy frequency. It, too should be used with caution.

On the physical level, orange can often help in cases of anemia, arthritis, diabetes, and congestion or rigidity of any kind. It has been used successfully in clearing up mucous and in breaking up calcium deposits. Constipation may be alleviated with an orange application.

On the mental and emotional level, orange can often lift people out of depression, and can bring self-confidence and courage to those with low self-esteem. It is an "outgoing" color and helps give motivation when needed. This color can be considered a freeing agent, as it can aid in loosening mental and emotional blocks, and can relieve repressed anxieties and fears. Orange can help, too, in giving stability to the character. "The effect of orange upon

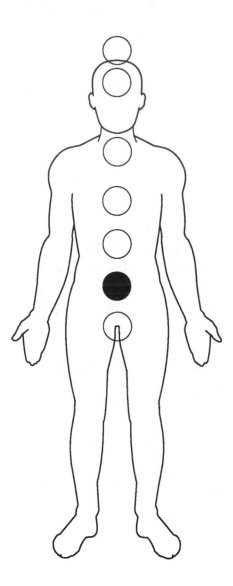

Figure 2. Orange relates to the sacral chakra (the second chakra), associated with the adrenal glands and the spleenic area. This center is activated by the orange part of pure white light.

the mentality is to aid the assimilation of new ideas and to induce mental enlightenment with a sense of freedom from limitations."[1]

The musical tone corresponding to orange is *D* in the middle octave, and chords in that key. The related glandular center is the spleenic area, that center in the body which receives the orange portion of Universal Light.

An individual on the orange path may be involved in work of a physical nature, but also he would be one who uses wisdom in whatever he does. Wisdom is one of the main characteristics of this color. These people would be very outgoing and prefer to work with groups rather than on a one-to-one basis. They would have (or *should* have if they are in tune with their basic key) a sense of self-respect and pride in accomplishments. The negative aspect of this energy would signify an over-emphasis on personal ego. This is something that positive-minded and success-oriented "orange" people must watch!

Understanding that we choose or agree to accept our path in life, we must then realize that the characteristics of this particular path need to be developed and used to full potential in this incarnation. Having our color around us, breathing it, wearing it frequently—all this will enhance our ability to perform as orange ray people. Other colors will and should be used when there is need for a certain energy vibration. No one color should ever be used to the exclusion of all others.

The next time you are faced with a stressful situation, try wearing something orange and have it around you to give courage and a feeling of self-worth. Then play some music with the uplifting and happy mood of orange and

---

[1]Roland Hunt, *The Seven Keys to Color Healing*, p. 57.

HUNGARIAN DANCE NO. 5 — *Brahms*

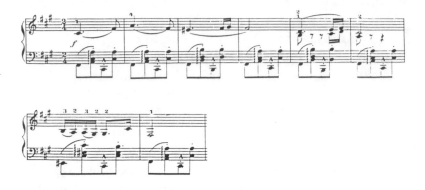

allow these energies to bring positive changes in your mental and emotional outlook.

In treating another, it should be remembered that counseling is usually indicated as a supplementary tool. When it seems advisable, counseling should be given if at all possible, as physical symptoms are almost always reflections of inner dis-ease. Treatment, as explained in the chapter on red, may employ colored light bulbs which are focused on the individual, localizing the light where there is a physical need.

Not only listening to related music, but also playing and/or singing can have great therapeutic benefits, as the whole person is then taking part in this healing treatment, and the very physical act of participation can loosen blocks and reduce tension.

Orange Music

Classical	New Age
Hungarian Dance no. 5 by Brahms	*Winterfall Music* by Paul Warner
Habanera from *Carmen* by Bizet	Jupiter Music from *The Planets* by Holst
Capriccio Espagnole by Rimski-Korsakov	*Eagle's Call* by Bruce Hurnow

Chapter Six

YELLOW

The gloriously beautiful yellow of the sun is the third color of the spectrum. Give yourself a sun bath by breathing, thinking, and visualizing a flow of yellow energy through your being.

As yellow is the third color of the spectrum, so it is also the third psychic center, relating to the solar plexus and the pancreas gland. This chakra is the seat of the emotions. It represents the "gut" level of our reactions, and is often referred to as the middle brain. Thoughts and emotions conceived in the mind are felt in the solar plexus. It is also considered the great brain of the nervous system. Yellow has a three-fold function: 1) it can stimulate the nervous system; 2) it deals with the emotions; 3) it activates the mental faculties.

There are physical energies within the yellow, but perhaps more importantly, there are vibrational frequencies within this color that strongly affect the mind and the emotions. Yellow should bring a happy, sunshiny outlook on life. At the same time—but perhaps under different conditions—this same color will stimulate the brain cells and will give the ability to study, analyze and to be the thinker.

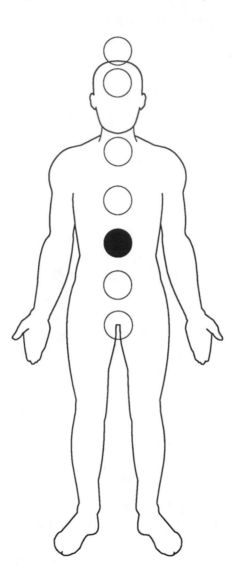

Figure 3. Yellow relates to the navel chakra (the third chakra), identified as the seat of our emotions, located in the area of the solar plexus and the pancreas gland.

People "coming in" on the yellow ray would be readers, students, and those who work best on a one-to-one basis. Mental work would be one of the main achievements. Care should be taken concerning emotional control, as this can sometimes present a problem for those on the yellow ray.

Whenever some very intense mental work is to be undertaken, wearing something yellow or being surrounded by this color can be very beneficial, because it actually stimulates the brain cells. Research has been done with a group of students with low IQ's. These students were separated into two different classes. One class was placed in a room with very drab walls and furniture, the other in a room with predominantly bright, cheerful colors, mostly yellow. Later the students were re-tested, and the group with mentally stimulating colors had raised their IQ level by a considerable degree. Those in the other group remained at the original low level of intelligence.

The music tone that correlates to yellow is C in the middle octave. As with the other colors and their repre-

ARABESKE *Schumann*

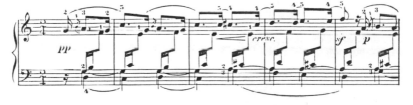

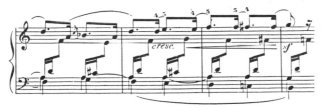

sentative keys, this note can be intoned, improvisations in the key of *E* can be played, or music in the yellow vibration can be received by listening to records or by actual participation with a musical instrument. Let the vibrations of this energy work for you. Listen and feel the response within you.

From a physical standpoint, yellow can be beneficial in alleviating constipation, arthritis, some sinus conditions, and problems of the liver and spleen.

On the mental level, this color can be applied to slow readers, and can be very effective in many cases of mental retardation.

Since the solar plexus area is the seat of the emotions, and since yellow is the color relating to this area, this could, then, be used in many instances in bringing emotional upheavals into better balance. As with other colors, yellow light may be projected to the solar plexus, and color breathing can also be very effective for healing the emotions.

Yellow Music

Classical	New Age
Arabeske by Schumann	*Lemurian Sunrise* by Warner
Fountains of Rome by Respighi	*Dawn* by Steven Halpern
Piano Concerto no. 26 by Mozart	*Kitaro Ki* by Kitaro

Chapter Seven

GREEN

Green, nature's master tonic, is the color of our planet at present. This color is representative of an evolutionary phase through which our world is presently progressing. It is said that planet Earth has already evolved through the first three paths — or the red, orange, and yellow levels — indicating physical and mental stages of growth. Now it is in the middle, or balancing, stage preparatory to the next step, which relates to blue, and indicates that Earth is readying itself to enter into a higher and more spiritual dimension. This color truly brings rest, tranquillity, and peace to the soul. It is needed at this time to bridge the gap between the more active or physical levels and the spiritual phases.

Green, being the middle of the spectrum with a blending of yellow on one side and blue on the other, is considered the great balancer. Therefore, it can often be used for healing in any situation when there may be a doubt as to the appropriate color energy needed. This green of nature can be wonderfully healing. To absorb its great energies, lie outside in the beauty of nature, feel and experience these natural vibrations.

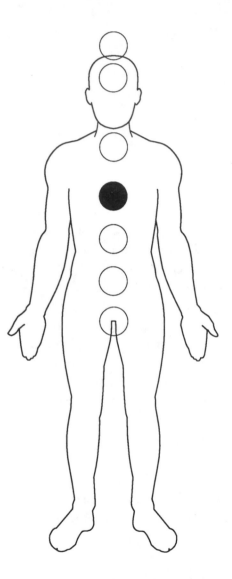

Figure 4. Green relates to the heart chakra (the fourth chakra). Both the color and the chakra have to do with the tranquillity and healing ability of the individual.

Other ways to experience green is to wrap yourself in a swatch of lovely, shimmering green cloth and then play a tape of, perhaps, Mendelssohn's *Spring Song*, the Neptune Music from the *The Planets*, or *The Fairy Ring*. Be aware of what this green energy does for you. Learn how to receive such energies into your being for balancing and centering. "Green" music as well as the color green can have wonderfully beneficial results for you as you allow it to flow through you.

Whenever you feel tense or irritable, pause a moment and see yourself enveloped in a bubble of green light and listen to related music. Much of the music of Scriabin, and particularly of Debussy, relates well to this energy because these composers were influenced greatly by Nature Spirits. New Age music also corresponds to the vibrations of nature, of growing things, and of waterfalls.

As mentioned in chapter one, green relates to the key of *F* and is the corresponding color to the heart chakra. This center exercises a strong influence on the circulatory system: thus, green, its color, can restore tired nerves and produce new energy. This is the color of growth and a renewing life. It can also be used as an aid in knitting bones and curing boils and ulcers. Green is such a soothing color that it can bring tranquillity to the nervous system.

Being a combination of blue and yellow, green works on an imbalance in blood pressure; yellow acts on the brain and refreshes and balances the pressure, while blue brings moderation and calmness. When stimulation and greater energy are needed, green is often preferable to a stronger color (such as red or orange) as these stronger colors might be too exhilarating for some individuals. Heart rhythms can often be normalized with green since it is such a balancer. It is interesting to note that chlorophyll,

CLAIRE DE LUNE

Debussy

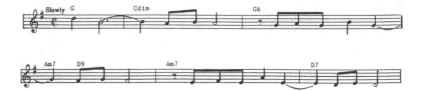

the green essence of nature, is now being used to balance heart action.

If you are one whose basic color is green, then you will probably have an innate healing ability and an affinity with the earth itself. For example, you might utilize herbs in your healing work. If you are a "green ray" person, you have a calm disposition and are able to reenergize yourself by walking barefoot in the grass or leaning against a tree to absorb its vibrations and energy.

Remember that green is the great balancer and can be used for almost any condition without harm. So when in doubt, try green.

He maketh me to lie down in green pastures. (Psalm 23:2)

I will lift up mine eyes unto the hills from whence cometh my help (Psalm 121:1).

Green Music

Classical	New Age
Melody in F by Ruben-stein	*Pan Flute* by Za Mir
	Ocean by Larkin
Violin Concerto in E Minor by Mendelssohn	*Fairy Ring* by Mike Rowland
Clair de Lune by Debussy	

Chapter Eight

BLUE

Blue relates to the key of G, and is the fifth color of the spectrum, relating to the fifth chakra—or the first of the three highest centers—the thyroid. This color represents spiritual awareness, a feeling of God-centeredness; it also signifies coolness, calmness, and inner peace. The blue person appreciates the beauty of the simplicities of life and nature.

If people need to look back into the past, this color will help lead them there, as it is a reflective color. It can also help people step ahead on the spiritual path. Religious aspirants are usually blue ray people, as truth, devotion, and dedication are qualities of blue. "It is through blue that we endeavor to penetrate the mysterious depths of the sea or the far reaches of the sky. So we say that God speaks to man of Infinity through the color blue."[1]

Blue is an electro-magnetic cooling color, and so is considered one of the best antiseptics available. This great cleansing color has proven to be effective in cases of skin eruptions. It is excellent for alleviating fevers and pain.

---

[1] Corinne Heline, *Color and Music in the New Age* (La Canada, CA: New Age Press, 1964), p. 41.

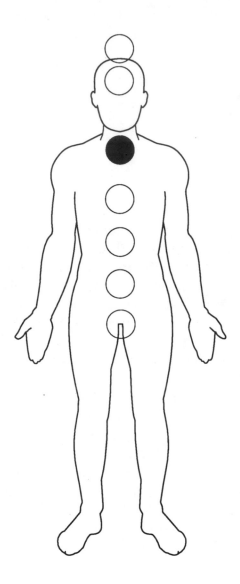

Figure 5. Blue relates to the throat chakra (the fifth chakra), which is the first of the three highest centers and hence represents spiritual awareness and inner peace.

Drinking solarized blue water can help cleanse internal infections. There are many other physical conditions that have been helped through the application of blue light, or the external and/or internal use of solarized blue water. (See chapter on techniques.) High blood pressure is often stabilized through the use of blue. Blue can be beneficial for sore throats, blood clots, acne, bladder infections, pneumonia, nausea, and burns.

Some cancerous growths can be dissolved with blue applications, as this color is considered a retardant and can prevent growth. Never use a stimulating color in the case of cancer, as that only energizes the condition rather than healing it.

Hyperactive people may often benefit from using blue frequently due to its calming effect. On the other hand, those who are lethargic would have a negative response to blue as it is too quiet and calming. Although blue has high spiritual vibrations, it would probably be too "low key" for people with low energy.

On a mental or spiritual level, this color can be of great benefit in bringing peace and calmness of spirit, and can be an aid in meditation. By absorbing these great spiritual vibes, the consciousness can be raised to a much higher degree.

Blue ray people would probably use the voice a great deal as this color relates well to the throat. These people might be singers, teachers, or lecturers. They should do everything in life with pure motivation, speaking only truth and desiring only to do God's will. This does not necessarily imply religious work, per se, but rather that people on the blue path have a motive to serve and to be honest in all dealings, regardless of the kind of work in which they might be involved.

AVE MARIA   *Schubert*

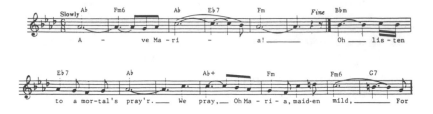

Something for blue people to watch is the coolness of blue. Often people on this ray appear cool and aloof because of their control and detachment. This is something to guard against so that balance is maintained.

If you want to meditate with blue, either wear something of this color, focus a blue light on yourself, or visualize this color enfolding your entire being. Then play some blue music and *allow* these beautiful vibrations to lift you into a higher state of consciousness. By exposing yourself to various vibrations, your whole being is changed as you receive these energy radiations.

It is interesting to note that blue is not only cooling but also brings a vibration of lightness. Try painting a heavy object with this color. Then lift it and you will actually feel that its weight has been reduced. This knowledge is used in many places such as warehouses where heavy boxes have to be lifted and moved constantly. When the boxes are painted blue, the workmen do not object nearly as much, as the weight appears to be lighter.

Blue can be used in various kinds of treatment. A person unknown to a color therapist asked for help on the phone. She wanted to remedy a skin condition. No medical treatment had alleviated the breaking and erupting of skin on the hands. The condition had existed for several years. The therapist prescribed the focusing of blue light over the hands for at least twenty minutes twice a day. This was done, and within two weeks the skin was completely clear. The hands could be immersed in water with detergent with no ill effect, and this was not possible a couple of weeks prior to this treatment. During this period no medication was used—only the blue light. The color treatments were given less often and soon discontinued.

A woman attending a color workshop asked for help with a fungus growth on the palms of both hands. During a group treatment, the blue light was used and the fungus almost completely disappeared on the left hand, while the right one, which was worse, did not show improvement. A blue light could be seen apparently flowing through the fingers of the left hand, as observed by everyone in the group.

The next morning, the woman came again to the workshop and showed the right hand which by then was 95 percent healed of the fungus. Another condition which this woman had not mentioned had also been remedied. For a period of about six months, this woman had not menstruated. However, the night following the blue treatment she resumed a normal flow. Although the blue can often *stem* the flow of blood, in this case the color acted as a cleansing agent, clearing out any blockage and purifying the hormones of the body, allowing for proper balance and adjustment.

Blue Music

Classical	New Age
Air on a G String by Bach *Ave Maria* by Schubert *The Swan* by Saint-Saens	*Divine Gypsy* (Instrumental arrangement of Yogananda's Cosmic Chants) *A Crystal Cave* (back to Atlantis) by Upper Astral Vocal Selection: *Be Still* by Rosemary Crow (United Research - Black Mt., N. C.)

Chapter Nine

INDIGO

Let the deep, mysterious beauty of indigo lead you into the inner recesses of your soul. Look into the indigo blue, visualize it filling the Third Eye, and let it draw you into a meaningful meditation.

This color is associated with the pituitary gland—or the Third Eye—and with the tone of *A* in the middle octave. As this chakra represents the intuitive sense, so indigo awakens inner knowing and alerts you to a realization of your responsibility in listening to and following this direction. If you are on this color path, you must find your answers to problems from your inner self rather than from analytical reasoning as does the yellow ray individual.

This color has a rather mysterious connotation because it leads into the depths of your being. It is a special color; its rich, deep shade tends to turn off the outside world for its emphasis is on the invisible within. Corinne Heline feels this color is not fully appreciated at the present. She says people are ". . . not fully aware of the power concentrated in the blending of the secondary col-

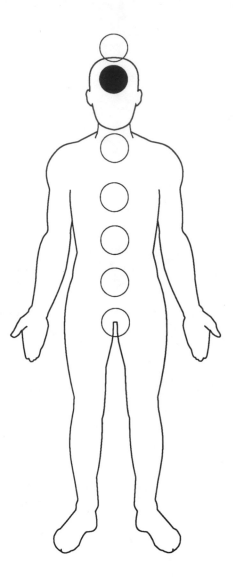

Figure 6. Indigo relates to the third eye chakra (the sixth chakra), which is the second of the three highest centers and is associated with the intuitive senses.

ors. A greater use of the Indigo Ray belongs to some future day."[1]

However, there are other authorities who do feel that we are ready to accept this healing ray, and it has proven to be very effective for many conditions that will be explained later in this chapter. Roland Hunt says, "Indigo, the Ray of the New Race consciousness, is his stabilizer, his Light-bearer; it is the Ray promoting our deeper seeing and feeling into the true realities of Life, to make them clearer to our united understanding.[2]

It is true that this color is one of very high spiritual vibration. It can help greatly in many situations, and yet may not be understood by the mass of humanity simply because of its highly charged energy.

Indigo, relating to the forehead area, may often be beneficial in conditions of the eyes, ears, and sinus. However, in many cases, particularly when the condition is chronic, a more stimulating color may be necessary to relieve congestion and blockage. In treating such a condition the therapist could then follow it up with the use of indigo.

Other imbalances frequently helped by the use of the indigo light are cataracts, nosebleeds, earaches, and dry coughing. This sixth ray color has a great influence on the mental and nervous structure. It can aid in healing epilepsy by eliminating negativity in the consciousness, lifting the individual to a higher and more stable awareness.

Intoning on *A* (indigo's note) can enhance the intuitive abilities, and music played in this key—or music that would be in this mood of ethereal quality—can readily raise spiritual awareness to a very high degree. As men-

---

[1] Corinne Heline, *Color and Music*, p. 42.
[2] Roland Hunt, *The Seven Keys to Colour Healing*, p. 92.

TRÄUMEREI   *Schumann*

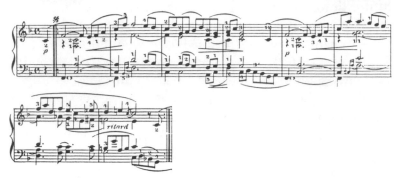

tioned in a previous chapter, blue, indigo, and violet are the three highest colors of the spectrum and correspond to the three highest chakras. Therefore, by the use of these highly vibrating colors, we are activated spiritually and become more aware of our divine nature.

Some people will find these last two colors (indigo and violet) are too high in vibrational frequency, so they cannot be absorbed with positive results. In such cases, it is suggested that blue be used first. These people should be allowed to grow gradually into a consciousness level where the higher vibrations can be more easily assimilated.

The color can be used in a variety of ways. For example, a cloth soaked in indigo solarized water can be placed on the eyes to give quick relief for inflammation. In a case of epilepsy, focus indigo light on the face and head to stabilize and aid in balancing.

To aid in meditation (for which indigo is especially helpful) have some of this color around and play music that relaxes you and lifts you into a spiritually meditative state.

For an interesting experiment, place a cloth or paper of indigo color on the area of the Third Eye. Try to *feel* this particular energy. Then do this with a different color and let your sensitivity feel the difference. If you do this experiment with different colors and on other parts of the body, you will soon learn to distinguish the differences in the various energies and vibrational frequencies of color. It will sharpen your intuitive sense and you will gradually become more sensitive to your inner spirit.

Indigo Music

Classical	New Age
Traumerei by Schumann	*Angel Love* by Aeoliah
Adagio Movement from Symphony no. 1 in C Minor by Brahms	*Inside* by Paul Horn
	Venus Music from *The Planets* by Holst
Poème for Violin and Orchestra by Chausson	

Chapter Ten

VIOLET

Violet, the seventh color of the spectrum, is a color of very high spiritual vibration. The application of this color and its appropriate music will greatly aid in reaching higher dimensions.

Violet is a regal color and people on this ray should be divinely centered; people who can lead others in lives of service and dedication to high ideals. The only sin on this path may be that of self-righteousness.

This color, as well as indigo blue and clear blue (the three highest colors on the spectrum) are all excellent for meditation.

Some of our greatest artists and musicians have been inspired by the use of the violet rays. It is said that Leonardo da Vinci meditated under violet rays falling through stained-glass windows. Wagner, when composing the Parsifal music, had violet drapes around him, thus absorbing these extremely high spiritual vibrations. Comte de St. Germain is said to have used these rays for healing purposes and for purifying gems.

The energies of the color violet, in addition to charging us spiritually, can also bring healing on a physical level in many instances. Epilepsy, for example, can often be allevi-

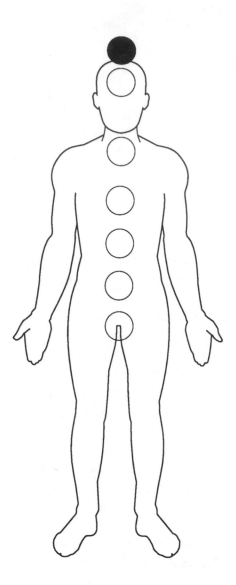

Figure 7. Violet relates to the crown chakra (the seventh chakra), which is the highest center of the human body. Both the color and the chakra are associated with our highest spirituality.

ated with the application of these vibrations. Also, cramps, kidney infections, and some cases of cerebrospinal meningitis have been helped with the use of violet. Some therapists recommend this color for healing mental disturbances. However, I feel that unless the individual is spiritually oriented, violet can be too stimulating—too high in spiritual vibrations—and its use could be devastating. Violet is as stimulating on a spiritual level as red is on the physical level. In such a case, blue might be applied, and then, perhaps, violet could be applied if and when the patient has become more sensitive to higher vibrations.

It is said that violet's "high rate of frequency is depressing to the moronic mind because its potencies are beyond its understanding; it is a stimulant mainly to the intuitive nature and has great inspirational effect on the highest human ideals."[1] "Violet is not suited to minds that are undeveloped, retarded or stunted, on account of its very high vibrational rate."[2]

The spiritual center corresponding to this color is located at the top of the head—the pineal gland—sometimes referred to as the Crown Chakra. This is often observed as having a center of gold and white light. Wisdom and spiritual vibrations reach us through this center, which in turn receives the energy from the universe. It is referred to in the East as the Thousand Petaled Lotus which opens its petals as we open up in a spirit of receptivity.

The musical tone relating to violet is *B* in the middle octave. If you play or intone on this note, try to be aware of the resonance in the Crown Chakra while playing or singing. As you intone on the violet note of *B*, it should

---

[1]Roland Hunt, *The Seven Keys to Colour Healing*, p. 103.
[2]S. C. J. Ouseley, *The Power of the Rays*, p. 79.

LIEBESTRAUM

Liszt

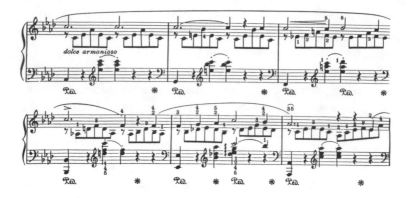

activate the pineal gland. So learn to tune in to this and become sensitive to the vibrations.

Violet is an excellent transmuting agent. It can be used to change a nervous or irritated state of mind into a calm and peaceful consciousness; it can also help to dispel insomnia. It is interesting to note that violet has germinating qualities and the violet light has been used successfully to cure baldness, even when no hair roots were remaining.

Cataracts have been helped by the application of the violet light. Also, a damp cloth soaked in violet solarized water (see chapter on techniques) can be placed over the eyes with beneficial effect.

Violet Music

Classical	New Age
Piano Concerto in B Minor by Tschaikovsky	*The Great Pyramid* by Paul Horn
Liebestraume by Listz	Neptune Music from *The Planets* by Holst
Gregorian Chants	*Eventide* by Steven Halpern

Chapter Eleven

PASTELS AND IRIDESCENCES

Pastel colors are a result of the normal spectrum colors being infused with white, and they have a beauty and delicacy all their own. Pastels may also be a combination of other colors, such as blending pink and yellow to make pastel peach. Using peach as an example, let's consider its relationship to the chakras and tones. On the keyboard, peach would relate to an interval of a major third – the C above middle C (pink) and E above the middle octave (light yellow). As for chakras, peach would correspond to a blending of the root chakra and the solar plexus, on a high vibratory level, displaying a somewhat different frequency than the relationship of pure red to the root chakra or spectrum yellow to the solar plexus. (Please refer to the chapters on red and yellow.)

Pastels are not better than the true spectrum colors, but they give a different focus, acting as a bridge between the spectrum (or the rainbow) and the iridescences that do give energies of a higher spiritual consciousness. People using pastel energies would think with the mind and heart. They differ from people who are more receptive to the iridescences because iridescences work entirely from an intuitive and spiritual nature, allowing influences from the cosmos to flow into them. There is a certain subtlety in pastel energies which might, it is felt, lead to that "in-between world," between waking and sleeping, where we are more receptive to intuitive leadings. Surrounding ourselves with pastels can help reach these other dimensions.

We experience lightness when working with these particular energies and this lightness may correspond with spatial and astral planes of thought. In addition, we could say that although pastels don't have the same strength as rainbow colors, their purpose may be in *accenting* the spectral colors and the iridescences, thereby adding to the energy and beauty of the whole. As soft, white clouds emphasize the beautiful blue of a clear sky, so may pastel shades accentuate the deeper and brighter colors.

Let us consider some examples of working with pastels. Red, when mixed with white, would give a rosy tone that signifies love. When it becomes an iridescent red, the energies are raised and it represents a divine, universal love. This color can be used by people needing this kind of love awareness. By adding more white, a softer pink is obtained, also indicating love, but on a more personal level. Peach was already mentioned as a combination of pink and light yellow. Then take a clear blue, add a bit of white, and see the beautiful pastel shade emerge. Work with these lovely pastels, and then with the spectrum colors. Become aware of the differences in your responses and determine when you might need a pure violet, for example, or when a lighter, pastel tone of this same color might be more helpful.

Iridescent colors—what are they? Webster says, "Iridescence is an interplay of rainbow colors." Think of them as dancing, shimmering lights—active like fireflies. We might see such an iridescence through a prism. However, it is also possible to have the iridescent effect of *one* color, although other colors may interweave.

If you take a piece of iridescent turquoise glass and hold it to the light, you will see not only the main color—turquoise—but a myriad of other colors, almost in the background as it were. You may see various shades of aqua and turquoise that will blend and give more life and vitality to the original color. This color can heal and invigorate the body, and is a powerful aid in your spiritual growth.

Try an iridescent green as opposed to a true green. You have increased the spiritual energy as well as adding a variety of colors and shadings. Buy some glass that has been treated with the iridescent colors, and/or get some fabric with iridescent threads woven in. Feel them, look at them, and put them close to your body. Test it out and you will be surprised at the difference in your response to them as compared with your feeling in response to pure spectrum colors. Observe the beauty of an iridescent golden yellow, the violet, and also white and silver. Wrap yourself in an electric, iridescent blue and see how it lights up your face, giving it additional spiritual light and vitality.

The true blue of the spectrum, as mentioned above, is always a great cleanser and purifier. So it is with the iridescent blue, only more so, and this frequency of blue will clear up imbalances in one's auric field. This can also be used for headaches. Iridescent blue may be applied for hypertension, always being aware of the spiritual receptivity of the individual whom you are treating. Another iridescent color that should be considered and used is fuchsia. When used on this high level, fuchsia may attract a Divine Soul to the individual.

As we apply these colors with the use of iridescent glass or fabric, we should visualize at the same time, for this creative action speeds up the effect and brings cosmic energies to the person being treated.

Iridescences reflect light, and when such a color is applied, there is an upward divine surge almost instantaneously. However, this is dependent on the individual's degree of evolvement. People with little spiritual awareness would undoubtedly not be receptive to these very high vibrations. On the other hand, people who are spiritually evolved would respond to the iridescent colors in a very positive and beneficial way. When giving treatments, the spiritual awareness needs to be evaluated first—by your own intuitive knowing and/or by the use of the pendulum, or by muscle testing (as explained in chapter thirteen).

In the past, there have been Temples of Healing that used the tools of color, music, gems, and herbs, and so will there be such temples again as we continue to reach upward in our spiritual quest. When we reach the right level, undoubtedly the iridescence of colors will be understood along with the great musical compositions. Then the methods of healing we are discussing here will be more widely taught and applied again.

Chapter Twelve

MANIFESTING UNIVERSAL ENERGIES WITH CRYSTALS

The word *crystal* is from the Greek "krystallos" (from "kryos") meaning "icy cold," and it was believed that quartz crystals were formed as a result of extremely hard frozen ice.

So what are crystals? Physically, they are fossilized water.[1] However, some crystals are formed when molten rock cools and mixes with various chemical combinations; others are formed when water or other solvents leave or "dries out." Today, crystals are made intentionally by both methods. Metaphysically, they are a part of the mineral kingdom that is expressing itself in an ordered fashion to become a greater part of the universal whole. Mathematically, for those who are interested, there is a calibration that equals the energy and frequency of the Great Pyramid, under and through which there is a great crystal.[2] So once again we see that all things are interconnected!

---

[1]Dael Walker, *The Crystal Book* (Sunol, CA: The Crystal Company, 1983), p. 13.
[2]Beverly Criswell, *Quartz Crystals* (Reserve, NM: Lavandar Lines, 1983), p. iv.

Some crystals originated many miles beneath the Earth's crust, under heat and pressure, in pools and veins. First, they were in a liquid form, but eventually they projected forth as a solid, bringing into manifestation the thought form that was first in Universal Mind—God. It was as if a print was produced out of the pure light of Spirit and this print penetrated the earth substance. These crystals, formed from within the Earth itself, are projected forth as solids. Crystal glass is not a solid, nor is it a true crystal.

As the minerals form, they must be in balance with the environment, but as the environment changes, so does the crystal formation. Isn't this true of all things, including our species? As a different "something" manifests in our surroundings, or in the growth process, necessary adjustments must be made to accommodate these changes. There is chemical activity in the atoms of crystals, and whenever a crystal breaks—exposing some of the interior layers—these atoms move around to adjust to the new situation.

> John Ruskin said of crystals, "They are wonderfully like human creatures . . . you will see crowds of them forced to . . . hurry . . . then you will find indulged crystals who have changed their minds and ways continually . . . been tired . . . been sick . . . and got well. . . ."[3]

Crystals are truly living entities; they have power and enjoy life deep *within* themselves. It has been said that crystals grow from the minerals in the Earth. One end always begins in earth matter, but the terminated end is pointed, and that end is usually used in directing the

---

[3]Paul E. Desantels, *The Mineral Kingdom* (New York: Madison Square Press, 1968), p. 69.

energy flow. The double terminated crystal doesn't come from the ground, but is conceived in a vaporized, gaseous type of "womb." The Herkimer Diamond is such a crystal.

The crystal is often referred to as a memory bank or a storage computer. Researchers who found and worked with the Crystal Skull, discovered in Central America, feel that when they tuned in to it (first, of course, being in tune with Universal Mind), facts of ages and civilizations were revealed to them. They literally read the records embodied in the crystal.

Indications are that thought forms can be projected into crystal, where they are stored to be brought forth when needed. Crystals apparently can hold not only thoughts but also vibrations of emotions, music, color and sound. These energies become available or are "readable" only to those who are in rapport with the Higher Self, and, thus, in tune with God. *All things are open to people who seek with the highest of motives.* According to one authority, "the spiral of energy that goes through a crystal, and the spiral of harmonics that is created by music or mantras correspond to one another by mathematical calibration. This is the harmonics and main basis for keeping the orchestration of the planets and galaxies in balance and harmony."[4]

When we think of storing thoughts and vibrations, is it not comparable to our absorbing a person's vibrations? We are often told to cleanse a crystal that another has touched, so that the energy of that person will be cleared from the crystal before we use it. This is based on the same concept that crystals can retain a vibrational energy—such as thought—which can then be felt or experienced by

---

[4]Beverly Criswell, *Quartz Crystals*, p. 13.

someone who has developed sensitivity to these vibrations.

The art of psychometry rests on this same concept. Holding an object that belongs to another person is thought to enable a psychic to pick up vibrations in feeling or in symbols that will reveal something about the owner of the object. Thinking of the Crystal Skull as a memory bank does not seem so incongruous when we remember that we, too, probably have experienced similar vibrational impacts. Have you not walked into a room and immediately felt quite comfortable? Or into another and felt a great urge to leave at once because something just didn't feel right? Perhaps you have picked up a crystal or some other object and have said, "This is just the perfect one for my friend." Rooms, objects, humans, and, of course, crystals do pick up vibrations and retain a certain amount of energy. So why might it not retain thought?

Consider the story of George Washington Carver. He communed with facets of nature—perhaps not the crystal but other living entities, namely the sweet potato and peanut! He "received" much useful information as to products that could be and were developed from these lowly form of life. These products were of help to mankind. He was able to tap into information stored in these pieces of energy because of his deep feeling for and belief in nature and God. There was a rapport between Carver and the sweet potato and peanut that enabled him to be receptive to the potential of this kind of energy growing from the Earth.

Let's bear all this in mind as we consider the crystal as a storage unit. As we become more and more attuned to the God-Self within—and to a particular crystal—we may be surprised at the feelings, pictures, and thoughts that are revealed to us. So talk and listen to your crystals and have fun!

And now, what can crystals do besides acting as a memory bank? They can be used for many healing needs, for meditation and for energy. First, let's remember that a thought is energy. If the thought, itself, tends toward balance and harmony, that thought will bring more balance and harmony when it interacts with a crystal. The crystal will increase the energy of the thought, good or bad. It does not discriminate. Comparable to our subconscious, it acts upon whatever we feed it.

As you use crystals on your energy centers, particularly the pineal and pituitary, your power to visualize improves. If you have trouble "seeing" when an object is mentioned, use a crystal, for it will help you. If you hear the words "red apple," do you instantly see it? If not, using the crystal on the third eye area should help this visual perception, and help your perception of auras, as well.

When you have thoughts or habit patterns that you wish to change, hold your crystal in your left hand (the receiving side) and project into your crystal computer the thought or habit pattern *you want to develop*. Do not give attention to the negativity that you wish to change. If you do this with sincere intent and with the highest motives, you should see positive results. It may be necessary to repeat the process several times. Be patient.

There is a great deal to learn and understand regarding the energies of crystals. When buying a crystal, you may want to check its energy level. You can measure this with a pendulum or with your own intuitive ability.

As we remember the old crystal radio sets, we can begin to appreciate some of the energy now being put to use in audio and visual equipment, in lasers and in space technology. "A tiny slice of quartz in a micro circuit increases an electrical signal such as a microphone."[5] Quartz is widely used for this purpose in many fields of modern electronics such as those mentioned above.

As we gain understanding of the tremendous energy of crystals, and as we decipher old records, it becomes clear that much of this subtle but real strength may have been used in erecting large buildings and perhaps in building the pyramids.

It would appear that crystal energy will enable us to establish better communication between the physical, mental, and spiritual worlds as we progress into the Aquarian Age. We have seen that it has enabled the radio to bring us sounds from the etheric waves. There is evidence that crystals store thoughts to be released when the correct time and environmental conditions are present. This makes communication upon many levels a distinct possibility for the future. We are already experiencing healing through this kind of energy, and undoubtedly crystals will be used in electronic devices for diagnosis and treatment. We have merely to understand and believe in the capabilities of crystals and then put them to use for individual and universal good.

By using crystals along with appropriate music and color, we have unlimited possibilities for spiritual growth, healing, and for deep insights into the higher dimensions of our world. It is also interesting to note that the use of music and color can aid in the growth of the crystal itself.

Another use of crystal energy is in revitalizing plants and water. Put a crystal in your drinking water, let it stand and then compare it with your regular "uncrystallized" water. You will sense a difference in taste, and you should

---

[5]Dael Walker, *The Crystal Book*, p. 13.

feel more energy after drinking crystallized water for a time. You might give your plants water that has absorbed this energy and then watch them grow! Just placing a crystal near your plant will also speed its growth.

It is essential to give your crystals good care. When you first acquire one, it should be cleared of any previous vibrations. To do this, immerse it in clear water, preferably with some salt. Authorities differ on the length of time that the crystal should be left in water. You might check this with your pendulum. A few hours would be advisable, or even overnight. If you put it in the sun, it would be cleansed and the sun would also charge it. It is helpful to do this from time to time as a general practice. Always, as with everything, your own positive visualization can do more to cleanse the crystal than anything else. See the pure light of Spirit flowing into the crystal, filling it with pure love and energy. Then keep it around you frequently, so it will pick up your own vibrations and be more responsive to your input.

It is often suggested that once the crystal is cleared and charged, it should be kept in a cloth of pure material such as velvet, cotton, or silk. Some authorities feel it should be kept in a black cloth to hold the energies within. My own feeling is that you and the crystal must get acquainted. Get to know the feel of it, try to sense its vibrations and then ask, either with the pendulum or from your own intuitive center, just what this particular crystal needs for its protection. As you work with it, having only the highest motives, you will learn how to treat it. If you plan to use it for healing, then it is best to keep your vibrations on it—and only yours. If, for any reason, someone else handles it, you can always clear it again before directing it to an individual or to yourself for healing purposes.

Crystals have electronic properties and, as the body is electronic in nature, you can relate very well to the crystal energy. Generally speaking, for healing you would hold the crystal in the left hand as this is the receiving side, and place the right hand on the pain area. This will allow the energy from the crystal to flow through to the right hand and infuse the pain area with its healing vibration. There are times, however, when you may feel you should place your left hand on the pain area, thus drawing out the imbalance, sending it to the right hand which holds the crystal. By sending the energy over your solar plexus area, you are able to let the crystal dissolve the negativity. There are still other situations in which you may be led to place the crystal, itself, directly over the pain. This has worked exceptionally well in some cases.

There are many techniques given for tuning in to and channeling this crystal frequency. It is always my feeling, however, that each of you has to find the method best suited to your own energy. Experiment with the crystal until you *feel* right in the way that you use it. Then, too, you may find that you develop different ways of using it for yourself in each specific problem, and in applying it for others. Visualize and meditate with the crystal. This is important, and always, if you are sincere and turn to the Highest for direction, you will be guided correctly. It is good, however, to remember that the left side is the receptive side, and the right is the out-going side. Also, keep in mind that it is not only the crystal energy, but also the thoughts that you put into the crystal that are fused into a single healing force.

There are many techniques suggested for using the crystal in meditation. One I like to suggest is just to sit quietly with the crystal in your left hand and feel yourself becoming part of it. Be receptive to the spiritual flow.

Then see yourself entering the crystal. Absorb the energy and look around, asking what is to be revealed to you. Then LOOK, LISTEN AND FEEL.

You may want to use the crystal as a pendulum to scan the body to find imbalances and bring the chakras into balance. Just hold the crystal as you would the pendulum and move your hand over the body. Try to be aware of the various sensations and any change in your response as you move it from one area of the body to another.

Experiment with your crystal. Become acquainted with the many different kinds of crystals and learn what each will do for you. See the bibliography for excellent references. Table 2 on pages 82–83 shows a few kinds of crystals and gems with their possible uses.

There are many gems, crystals, and minerals that are worthy of your investigation and experimentation. Do enjoy this "tool" for stones have already been an aid to mankind. They will provide more energy as we understand and use these natural energies properly.

We talk about the use of crystals in this "new age." Every age is a new age, and let us not forget that in early Egypt "new age," crystals and gems, as well as color and music, were understood and used for healing and energy builders on a regular basis.

> One phenomenon that still excites superstitious speculation, and must have puzzled earlier men to the point of terror, is a meteorite. The ancient Jews held these mysterious objects in special reverence. They called them 'Beth-el' which means 'House of God,' because they believed that the fallen fragments carried the blessings of God directly from Heaven.
>
> These early Jews added other superstitions to mineral lore; among them was a story that one of

Table 2. Uses for Crystals and Gems.

Stones	Healing Uses
Clear quartz	Used as an overall body energizer.
Smokey quartz	Helpful when grounding is needed.
Green quartz	A body balancer.
Pink Rose and Citrine	Both can be used to balance the body and the four highest chakras.
Neutral Citrine (light orange to brown)	A balancer for the three lowest chakras.
Tumbled citrine (golden color)	Stimulates the crown chakras.
Opal	A rather mystical stone. It picks up the atmosphere round it and also reflects the person wearing it, especially if the individual is a Libra.

King Solomon's rings was set with a stone of such peculiar power that he had only to gaze at it to know everything he needed to know at a given moment.[6]

Gems have long been associated with our religious and cultural history, and they have been and still are connected with the signs of the zodiac. Twelve gems were worn on the breastplates of the High Priests of old, relating to the twelve months of the year and the zodiac. In King Solomon's Temple, gold and silver were used. Silver

---

[6]Paul E. Desantels, *The Mineral Kingdom*, pp. 12–13.

Table 2. (continued).

Stones	Healing Uses
Opal (cont.)	Wear it at different times and observe how it changes your emotions and/or other physical conditions. This stone can also help to open the third eye.
Lapis Lazuli	Good as a stabilizer and for clearing the mind. Often used in the Priests' breastplates.
Flourite	A good conductor of energy. Very helpful in meditation.
Emerald	Good for the eyes. Is an antidote to poison. Definitely a healing stone.
Silver	A stabilizer. Relates to the moon and space.
Gold	Magnifies feelings.
Copper	Helps with a copper deficiency, and with arthritis and other pains.

was considered to have a subjective quality as it was believed that silver was gold with its sun's rays turned inward. It represented the purified and reborn human nature. Gold signifies spirituality, and in the Temple it was placed over wood, indicating the spiritual nature glorifying the physical person.[7]

Crystals, gems, and minerals arc, indeed, marvelous examples of God's magnificent creation. They are living and growing entities. Colors and our perception of them

---

[7]Manly P. Hall, *Secret Teachings of All Ages*, p. cxxxv.

have evolved as we have evolved. In other words, as human beings developed, we began to perceive more objects and to distinguish between colors. So it is with the planet and everything on it, such as minerals and crystals. They evolve, take form, and grow, as we grow into ever greater spiritual awareness.

Chapter Thirteen

TECHNIQUES

As we develop our awareness and understanding of the properties of tones and colors, we must learn the "how-to" of applying these energies to bring healing to the physical, emotional, and spiritual bodies. It is most important that we properly evaluate the individual whom we are treating. We are each unique in our own way. Therefore, our needs are different and our responses vary accordingly. So we must learn to check out each problem and then apply the tools that will help in that particular situation.

When we prepare to give a color/music treatment, we should first find the person's basic color ray. This will give us an idea of that person's path—the strengths and weaknesses. Taking that into consideration along with understanding the specific problem, we can then determine the proper tones and colors to use.

One way to find the color path is to use the muscle test. Have the patient sit or stand with his or her stronger arm perpendicularly extended in front of the body, while the other hand holds a sample color. The therapist should then ask mentally for the right color while pushing down on the arm at the wrist; the patient should try to resist. If the person is able to resist the pressure on the stronger arm, it is indicative of a positive reaction to the color. If the patient is unable to resist the downward push, it shows a negative response—meaning that this color is not good for that person.

This kind of muscle test can be used to test many other things besides color, for example, to test food for which you may be allergic. You can also use the test to see what musical notes are best for you. However, once you have found the correct color or tone, then you would know that the related tone or color (as explained in Table 1 on pages 4–5, and in the chapters on colors) would have comparable vibrations. Both the related tones or colors should be used together to give additional strength.

Another way to determine the basic color is with the pendulum. Any lightweight object, such as a ring or small piece of jewelry that can be fastened to a string (or chain) and can be balanced, may be used as a pendulum. However, the higher quality the pendulum, the better the results—a crystal, for instance, or a good metal is excellent as a pendulum. However, a needle and thread will work for you too! There are a lot of pendulums that you can buy; try the local metaphysical bookstore.

When you have your pendulum ready, hold it over your left hand (the receiving side) to acquaint the pendulum with your vibrations and to start the action. Then, when it starts moving, ask it to show you your "yes" and "no" signals. You may have to work with this a while in order to understand it, and for the pendulum to become used to picking up your vibrations. Always remember that the *motive* with which you use this tool is important. The energy from your own Higher Self (not magic in the pendulum) is what works for you as a spiritual aid. Ask only for truth and evaluate carefully, knowing that you are still a human channel. Recognize that the more spiritual your consciousness is, the greater will be your receptivity to truth.

If you wish, find the tone first, then relate it to its corresponding color. To do this, play various notes on a musical instrument and try to determine which tones or keys evoke a deep response within you. This requires an honest searching into your inner self. The difficulty is that you may respond to a specific color or tone at a given time because of a particular need at that moment. This color/tone may or may not show your path for this entire incarnation. It is advantageous, therefore, to have another person, who can be more objective, do this for you. It may also be advisable, when checking for the note, to test at different times under various circumstances and/or at different times of day in order to eliminate external influences.

Do understand that these techniques are to be used, not only to find the color path, but also to determine the "tools" needed for any treatment, to determine the length of time required, and to measure the effect of these applications.

When a basic color is assigned, many people tend to reject it, expressing dislike for that particular color. This *usually* indicates that these people do not accept the qualities represented by that particular color ray. For example, a young woman came to the color therapist for a color analysis. Her basic color was found to be green. She never liked green, but lately had been drawn to green in spite of her previous dislike for it. It was explained that green represented healing qualities, among other things. At this point the client stated that she was a nurse and recently had noticed that the patients with whom she worked were responding to her care more than was normally the case with nursing per se. She had previously been afraid of this kind of in-depth healing and had not understood the spiritual aspect of it. It is interesting to note that as she began to accept the spiritual healing quality within herself, she was also beginning to like this color. Many times we fight our natural path, but as we begin to accept that which we truly are, then everything begins to fall into place. It's called the divine order!

The methods of applying color and music for healing are varied and depend a great deal not only on the therapist's preference but, most importantly, on the client's level of receptivity. With some people, pure visualization of a color may be sufficient and, perhaps, may even give forth a greater vibrational energy than when you send color by using a physical tool. On the other hand, some people may not realize the power of visualization, and its very important to *see* the physical application of the technique.

Some of the physical aids that you can use are colored light bulbs, colored gels that are made to be used in a slide projector, and solarized water. If you work with the light bulbs, the wattage of the bulb is not as important as the color itself, but a 75 to 100 watt bulb is recommended. The important thing to remember in any kind of treatment is that the tool (as well as the therapist) are only channels through which these vibrational energies may be received.

The light bulb should be in a lamp that can be adjusted to focus over a specific area on the body that needs the healing. Sometimes, however, the light should be focused over the head for an overall application. In cases of poor circulation, a stimulating color (to be determined individually, as I mentioned earlier) should be applied to the base of the feet where there are nerve endings, as well as to the spine. In severe cases, use the color at least twice a day for fifteen minutes to a half hour.

The length of time for treatment can be ascertained either by the client's own response, by the use of the pendulum, checking with the muscle test before and after treatment for energy levels, or by the therapist's intuitive knowledge. Usually some response is felt almost immediately, such as vibrations in the body, various kinds of activity, and perhaps some warmth or coolness. Some people may sometimes feel irritated or relaxed after treatment. This depends on the condition being treated. The irritation or the relaxation are both signs to determine whether treatment should be continued or discontinued at that point. In many cases, people will have a delayed reaction to the color, so don't wait until some response is felt, as people are unique. The therapist must know each individual as an individual and not categorize people or their reactions.

Another therapeutic use of color comes from working with solarized water. To prepare this, put water into a *glass* container of the color desired. Place it (covering only the top) in the direct sunlight for a minimum of two hours. This water may then be drunk or applied externally, depending on the circumstances. For example, you can drink blue solarized water to alleviate kidney infections, bladder problems, or any internal inflammation. If you drink red solarized water, it can greatly aid in energizing circulation and can act as a blood builder. Use the applications of water along with light treatments.

If you drink yellow solarized water (or orange, depending on the severity of the condition, as orange is stronger than yellow) it is an excellent cure for constipation. Blue solarized water can help the opposite condition—that of diarrhea.

Experiment with this concept. Try putting water into several different colored glass containers. Then slowly taste each one. As you continue to do this, you will develop a sensitivity toward the different color tastes.

Visualization is another tool for receiving color energies, as the power to visualize is a very creative one. Try "seeing" a bubble of a color needed around yourself. As you think, as you visualize, you do create the energy of that particular color. You bring forth whatever your mind images. You may do this for another person also, by visualizing for him or her. Concentrate on the image and you will maintain that vibrational energy.

When you are giving an application of color, also use music that will have the proper correlation with the particular color being used. Play records or tapes that apply to the color or chant and/or intone a specific note.

Toning can be done on the AUM or OM sound on your own basic note, or you can use the specific tone needed for a particular ailment. In a group, the harmony produced by everyone intoning on whatever note they choose can be extremely inspiring and healing. The dissonances that you might expect turn into beautiful harmonies!

In certain situations, it can be much more beneficial to use a single note rather than a full selection with various harmonies and rhythms. For example, in treating a sinus condition, it would be more effective to intone one note, probably D in the middle octave for this tone gives the energy required to break up the congestion. Instead of intoning, this note could also be played on an instrument or a pitch pipe. At the same time, the orange light (relating to D) should be focused directly on the sinus area. In this way, the energies are more concentrated than if an array of colors and tones were used. Using both modalities—color and music—will increase the vibrational energies.

Another way of intoning is to start with the AH sound, then going to OH, then to OOOO and finally to EEEE. The idea is to start at the bottom with a groan, letting out all tension, frustration, and anger. Keep moving the sound up and down until you find a tone that resonates with you. It may or not resonate on your special key note, but you may feel a response somewhere that could indicate an imbalance in that spot. In that case, stay with the tone until you feel a leveling off of the discomfort. Continue raising the tone slowly, all the time being aware of your feelings.

Toning can balance the energies and bring the mind and body into one unified whole. Clairvoyants have watched people when toning and have seen the energy go to an area that needs healing or balancing. When toning, don't force it. Just let it go, and let the tone find its own level.

There are times when it will be better to encourage people's participation in the music through singing or playing an instrument. The very act of singing does of necessity open them up and releases tension. Both playing and singing aid creativity and self-expression. However, it must be understood that if some people have been accomplished performers and cannot do well now, this may prove to be frustrating rather than beneficial. On the other hand, if they have been deprived of musical expression, then the chance to play or sing again may be just the therapy needed to "open the doors." Once again, the individual must be properly assessed as to needs and functional ability at the time of treatment, as not everyone is alike.

You must also consider that people may react in a positive way to one color or piece of music one day, but at another time they may have a very different response to the same treatment. This is because people are constantly changing moods, states of mind, and physical health. Therefore, their needs and responses may differ from time to time. The need to constantly evaluate the people with whom you are working cannot be emphasized enough. It is very essential in any treatment. It is also interesting and important to know that the effectiveness of any treatment of this nature may differ with the one-to-one relationship of therapist and client. This is due to the exchange of energies inherent in this type of healing work.

Be very aware of the proper correlation of music and color. For instance, people would not want to listen to Venus music from *The Planets* (ethereal sounds) and at the same time be surrounded by red vibrations!

Some of the techniques for applying music have been explained in the chapter entitled "You Are a Musical Instrument." The healing qualities of classical and new age music have been explained earlier. It is necessary to understand that hard rock music can only have a destructive effect to the healing process.

There are situations, however, when harsh, loud and/or discordant music *may* have a positive result. This happens when you find a certain rigidity in the body or emotions. In this case, music that would shock *might* be used to advantage. Use this music with extreme caution and for only a very short period of time. This type of music would be used for the purpose of loosening blockages. For people with great hostility and aggressive tendencies, beating on drums could bring relief. In these situations, however, when loud, strong music and drum beating might be applied, it should *always* be followed with a treatment of the personal basic color and tone for balancing and quieting. Green or blue-green can also be used to balance almost any situation, even if it is not the individual's basic color.

When you are working with hyperactive children, you can pick up their uneven rhythm or spastic movements on the piano or any instrument (if you can improvise) and thus gain rapport with the child. Then bring them to the point of calmness with appropriate music and color.

Bear in mind that our favorite color may not necessarily be the one representing our path in life. We often choose colors or music because of a need at the moment. In many cases this may signify an intelligent use of color or music. For instance, we may desire to wear red during a certain period of our lives. At the same time, we may be drawn to strong, rhythmic music. Perhaps, at the time, we are in need of physical energy. Being drawn to red does not necessarily imply that it is the best color/music path for our entire life. At another time, we may choose to wear black and may, at that point, like music of a somber or sad quality. This might indicate a period of turning within and this turning could be positive or negative. It could even indicate a hiding of sorts. For more information, refer to the chapter on Colors and the Aura.

A young woman who had been in a mental institution was referred to a halfway house where color and music therapy were used. This woman dressed consistently in dull beige or brown. When asked for her favorite color, those were the ones she chose. This was a definite indication of her insecurity, and her need to hide from the world. Dull, dark colors tend to bring the quality of concealment. To suggest that she, at that point, wear a bright red dress would have produced a shock to her entire system. Rather, she was offered the opportunity to wear various colored scarves as a means of developing a more positive outlook, meanwhile gradually introducing brighter and more colorful clothes, along with happy music. She was receptive to these ideas and expressed her liking for the colors and, therefore, she accepted this treatment. The gradual change is much more healing and positive than an abrupt shift from depression and fear to great joy and extroversion, and vice versa.

The clothing we wear, the colors in our homes and the music in our lives can contribute to a healing, happy atmosphere, or a destructive and depressing one. When we understand the vibrations of the various colors, then we can choose what we will wear to enhance our energy, to lift us out of depression, or to provide us with mental stimulation. We can experiment with colors and work with a variety of shades and hues—and give the same thought to the colors in our homes. Our work areas do well with red or oranges, mental work needs yellow, and the quieting colors would be indicated for the areas where we want to relax.

One more aspect to consider is that of recognizing when we use one color almost exclusively. This is an indication of imbalance and is a sign to look deeply within as to the reasons. Anything carried to excess signals a problem area. Moderation and balance are the key words!

As you experiment with different colors and various types of music and instruments, be aware of the difference in energy as well as in your spiritual and emotional outlook. Many changes will take place as you explore your feeling reaction to the spectrum.

Breathing is another great technique for bringing color vibrations into your being. Take deep breaths as you SEE the color you want, and FEEL the flow as you breathe in deeply and slowly, allowing these vibrations to enter your body, mind, and emotions. Do this several times, repeating it often, and you will begin to be more and more aware of your response to these color frequencies.

Color and music are excellent tools for healing on all levels. Take time to experiment with these techniques and let these energies lift you into a new dimension of living.

Chapter Fourteen

CONCLUSION

It is hoped that this book will have opened doors for a greater understanding of the wonderful, healing benefits of music, color, and crystals. This is not a new science but, hopefully, this will be a new adaptation of an age-old philosophy and modality. Every religion has an exoteric and an esoteric meaning, and color and music have a physical, or outer, interpretation and also an inner or in-depth significance.

There are many, many spiritually inspiring musical compositions which can, with the additional help of color, raise our consciousness to the level of the Masters. The works of various composers may activate different parts of the body, may harmonize the emotions and lift spiritual awareness. We have within us that ability to feel, to sense, and to become aware of these subtle but very powerful energies. Corinne Heline has quoted Rudolf Steiner as saying, "You have your eyes, you have your ears: look with your eyes on the things of Nature; hear with your ears what goes on in Nature; the spiritual reveals itself through color and through tone; as you look and listen you cannot help feeling how it reveals itself in these."[1]

Opinions vary, of course, in evaluating composers. the following relationships are among those which have been suggested: Bach, Beethoven and Mozart may aid in integrating the elements of the physical body, and Bach, Beethoven and Wagner may be considered the forerunners of the divine music of the future. For the purpose of searching within self, much of the music of Tchaikovsky is suggested, and for reflecting into the past, Debussy, Mahler and Chopin. Choral music of a high caliber often brings emotional release and spiritual uplift. These are merely suggested for your study. Each one of us must find that to which we can relate in a positive, healing way. We must each develop an inner awareness as to what music and color is saying to us individually; only when we respond with a depth of feeling can we gain maximum benefit from these subtly spiritual tools. As we try to harmonize with beautiful musical and inspiring rainbow colors, we should have a sense of expectancy and a feeling of openness, a readiness to receive. Let the great possibilities within color and music inspire us to further explorations.

Children can be helped immeasurably by being exposed to a variety of colors from their youngest years. The idea of having classrooms painted in the colors of the rainbow, each classroom in *one* color to exemplify stages in the child's growth has been successfully used in the Rudolf Steiner and Waldorf schools. The concept is that "when the child's education is complete he will have had the experience of 'living,' stage by stage, through all the

---

[1]Corinne Heline, *Color and Music in the New Age*, p. 71.

seven colors, which are an image of his own development."[2]

Industries, schools, and hospitals are beginning to recognize the value of color and music. They are accepting and utilizing these concepts more than ever before. However, "While music therapy has been proven to be of great value in hospitals—where it is often used in conjunction with recreational therapy—it is still handicapped by the absence of intuition, spontaneity and spirituality, three essential elements in body harmonization with its cosmic counterpart."[3]

It has been said that as our color experiences become more intimate, we grow closer in attunement with God. So it is with music. The proper use of color and music lifts us beyond the material world into a place that is more universal. Someday color and music will be the tools, not only for healing, but for communication with other people and hopefully with those in other worlds. Physical science, medical science, and the spiritual sciences are rapidly reaching a point of mutual understanding, and this gives great hope and expectations for this wonderfully creative age in which we live.

---

[2]Goethe, *Goethe's Theory of Color* (Sussex, England: New Knowledge Books, 1970), p. 35.
[3]Horatio Costa, "New Age Music," p. 67.

Glossary

Archetype: the original pattern, or the ideal, of your Higher Self; the blueprint of your "I AM."

Astral: the first subtle (invisible) but true body of the human being next to the physical; relates to the astral plane in the spirit world. The astral body is the seat of the emotions.

Aura: from the Greek "avra," meaning "breeze." Light energy, usually seen in colors which emanate from the physical and subtle bodies. For those who can see this, it can be a valid diagnostic tool.

Chakra: a Sanskrit word meaning "wheel." A psychic center of energy in the etheric body, superimposed over the seven main glandular centers in the physical body.

Clairaudience: clear (inner) hearing.

Clairsentience: clear (inner) knowing.

Clairvoyance: clear (inner) seeing.

Coccygeal: small, triangular bone at the base of the spine.

Cosmic Consciousness: universal, etheric, all-knowing consciousness; God-Mind.

Devic: devic kingdom refers to the angelic beings as well as to the nature spirits and elements.

Emanation: an outpouring; flowing forth.

Esoteric: a deep or inner (spiritual) interpretation of anything; a symbolic meaning behind words.

Etheric (Etheric body): a duplicate or "carbon copy" of the physical body, immediately next to the physical, but not a true or separate body as is the astral. Also refers to the "ethers" in the atmosphere—a substance into which impressions are made, i.e., the Akasha (the Cosmic Library) where records of events are stored.

Exoteric: outer, superficial, literal.

Iridescence: an interplay of rainbow colors.

Occult: hidden, secret.

Pineal: small, cone-shaped gland in the middle of the brain.

Pituitary: small, oval endocrine gland in the "third eye" area of the brain.

Psychic Centers: please refer to "chakras."

Spectrum: series of colors arranged according to their respective wave lengths by the passage of pure light through a prism; spectrum colors as seen in the rainbow.

Subtle bodies: invisible to the physical eye because of their vibrations being higher than those of physical bodies. they are visible to the trained clairvoyant.

Bibliography

Babitt, Edwin. *Principles of Light and Color*. Hyde Park, NY: University Books, 1967.

Baer, Randall N., and Viki Baer. *The Crystal Connection*. San Francisco: HarperCollins, 1987.

The Bible. King James Version. Nashville: Thomas Nelson, Inc., 1976.

Birren, Faber. *Color Psychology and Color Therapy*. Hyde Park, NY: University Books, 1965.

Blavatsky, Madame. *The Secret Doctrine*. Pasadena, CA: Theosophical University Press, 1952.

Cayce, Edgar. *Searchlight*. Virginia Beach, VA: A.R.E. Press, Dec. 1960, Dec. 1965.

Cornelio, Marie Wiliams. *Gemstones and Color*. West Hartford, CT: The Triad Publishing Co., 1985.

Costa, Horatio. "New Age Music, Cosmic Sounds and the Music of the Spheres," *The American Theosophist*. (May/June 1989), p. 63.

Criswell, Beverly. *Quartz Crystals*. Reserve, NM: Lavandar Lines, 1983.

Desantels, Paul E. *The Mineral Kingdom*. New York: Madison Square Press, Grosset & Dunlap, 1968.

Goethe, J. W. von. *Goethe's Theory of Color*. Sussex, England: New Knowledge Books, 1964.

Hall, Manly P. *Secret Teachings of All Ages*. Los Angeles: Philosophical Research Society, 1975.

Heline, Corinne. *Color and Music in the New Age*. La Canada, CA: New Age Press, 1964.

_____. *Healing and Regeneration through Music*. Santa Barbara, CA: J. F. Rowny Press, 1933.

Hodges, Doris M. *Healing Stones*. Hiawatha, IA: Pyramid Publishers, 1961.

Hunt, Roland. *Seven Keys to Colour Healing*. Saffron Walden, England: C. W. Daniel, 1971.

Isaacs, Thelma. *Gemstones, Crystals & Healing*. Black Mountain, NC: Lorien House, 1984.

Krippner, Stanley, and Daniel Rubin, eds. *The Kirlian Aura*. Garden City, NY: Anchor Books, 1974.

Ostrander, Sheila, and Lynn Shroeder. *Psychic Discoveries Behind the Iron Curtain*. Englewood Cliffs, NJ: Prentice-Hall, 1970.

Scott, Cyril. *Music: Its Secret Influence*. Wellingborough, England: Aquarian Press, 1933.

Walker, Dael. *The Crystal Book*. Sunol, CA: The Crystal Company, 1983, p. 13.